Words of Love II . . .
The Romance Continues

Also edited by
Tina Reed

WORDS OF LOVE

WORDS OF
LOVE II . . .

The Romance Continues

EDITED BY
TINA REED

A PERIGEE BOOK
New York

*Once again, the author wishes to thank
Bertha, David, Bob and Nancy.*

.

Perigee Books
are published by
The Berkley Publishing Group
200 Madison Avenue, New York, NY 10016

Library of Congress Cataloging-in-Publication Data

Words of Love II . . . the romance continues /
edited by Tina Reed.
p.   cm.
ISBN 0-399-51877-0
1. Love—Quotations, maxims, etc.   I. Reed, Tina.
II. Title: Words of love 2.
III. Title: words of love two.
PN6084.L6W662   1994
808.88′2—dc20   93-50874 CIP

Cover design by Terrence Fehr
Cover photo © by H. Armstrong Roberts, Inc.
Printed in the United States of America
1   2   3   4   5   6   7   8   9   10

This book is printed on acid-free paper.
∞

Words of Love II . . . The Romance Continues

*W*hen you love someone all your
saved-up wishes start coming out.
—*Elizabeth Bowen*

·

When you spice a dish with love, it'll
tickle every palate, I do believe. Not a
thing can be either salt or sweet without
a dash of love: it will turn gall, bitter
though it may be, to honey—an old
curmudgeon to a pleasing and
polished gentleman.
—*Plautus*

·

We went to Sunday school, public
school from the fifth grade through high
school, graduated in the same class and
marched down life's road together. For
me she still has the blue eyes and golden
hair of yesteryear.
—*Harry S. Truman*

*W*herever she is there is sun
And time and a sweet air
Peace is there
Work done
—*Archibald MacLeish*

.

Things are beautiful if you love them.
—*Jean Anouilh*

.

Love me Sweet, with all thou art,
Feeling, thinking, seeing;
Love me in the lightest part,
Love me in full being.
—*Elizabeth Barrett Browning*

.

A woman unsatisfied must have luxuries.
But a woman who loves a man would
sleep on a board.
—*D. H. Lawrence*

*I*t seems to me that the coming of love is like the coming of spring—the date is not to be reckoned by the calendar. It may be slow and gradual; it may be quick and sudden. But in the morning, when we wake and recognize a change in the world without, verdure on the trees, blossoms on the sward, warmth in the sunshine, music in the air, we say spring has come.
—*Edward G. Bulwer-Lytton*

.

In literature as in love, we are astonished at what is chosen by others.
—*André Maurois*

.

Only choose in marriage a woman whom you would choose as a friend if she were a man.
—*Joseph Joubert*

A man knows his companion in a long
journey and a little inn.
—*Thomas Fuller*

·

As you are woman, so be lovely:
As you are lovely, so be various,
Merciful as constant, constant as various,
So be mine, as I yours for ever.
—*Robert Graves*

·

Love, I find, is like singing. Everybody
can do enough to satisfy themselves,
though it may not impress the neighbors
as being very much.
—*Zora Neale Hurston*

·

Love is meat and drink, and a blanket
to boot.
—*American Proverb*

$\mathcal{T}$here is no place like a bed for
confidential disclosures between friends.
Man and wife, they say, there open the
very bottom of their souls to each other;
and some old couples often lie and chat
over old times till nearly morning.
—*Herman Melville*

.

The two divinest things this world
      has got,
A lovely woman in a rural spot!
—*Leigh Hunt*

.

It is not time or opportunity that is to
determine intimacy; it is disposition
alone. Seven years would be insufficient
to make some people acquainted with
each other, and seven days are more than
enough for others.
—*Jane Austen*

*L*ove affairs have always greatly
interested me, but I do not greatly care
for them in books or moving pictures. In
a love affair I wish to be the hero, with
no audience present.
—*Edgar Watson Howe*

.

Any man has to, needs to, wants to
Once in a lifetime, do a girl in.
—*T. S. Eliot*

.

I always say beauty is only sin deep.
—*Saki (H. H. Munro)*

.

Ask me no more whither do stray
The golden atoms of the day;
For in pure love heaven did prepare
Those powders to enrich your hair.
—*Thomas Carew*

*W*omen complain about sex more often
than men. Their gripes fall into two
major categories: 1) Not enough.
2) Too much.
—*Ann Landers*

.

Love is anterior to life,
Posterior to death.
—*Emily Dickinson*

.

Jenny kiss'd me when we met,
　　Jumping from the chair she sat in;
Time, you thief, who love to get
　　Sweets into your list, put that in!
Say I'm weary, say I'm sad,
　　Say that health and wealth have
　　　miss'd me,
Say I'm growing old, but add,
　　Jenny kiss'd me.
—*Leigh Hunt*

I wished a companion to lie near me in the starlight, silent and not moving, but ever within touch. For there is a fellowship more quiet even than solitude, and which, rightly understood, is solitude made perfect. And to live out of doors with the woman a man loves is of all lives the most complete and free.
—*Robert Louis Stevenson*

.

I knew it was love, and I felt it was glory.
—*Lord Byron*

.

The marriage urge has been know to sneak up on many couples who *thought* they were happily living in sin but then found themselves talking joint tax returns and honeymoons in Megève.
—*K. T. and Otis Maclay*

*W*ould I were free from this restraint,
  Or else had hopes to win her;
  Would she could make of me a saint,
  Or I of her a sinner.
        —*William Congreve*

.

You must believe me when I tell you
that I have found it impossible to carry
the heavy burden of responsibility and to
discharge my duties as King as I would
wish to do without the help and support
        of the woman I love.
  —*Edward VIII (Duke of Windsor)*

.

    Beautiful is she, this woman,
    As the mountain flower;
    But cold, cold, is she,
    Like the snowbank
    Behind which it blooms.
          —*Haida Song*

When I was one-and-twenty
  I heard a wise man say,
  Give crowns and pounds and guineas
  But not your heart away.
      —*A. E. Housman*

.

From my observation, marriage turns
  men to mush and bliss to blahs.
      —*Jeannie Sakol*

.

To write a good love letter, you ought
to begin without knowing what you
mean to say, and to finish without
knowing what you have written.
      —*Jean-Jacques Rousseau*

.

The extreme form of passionate love
  is secret love.
      —*Japanese Proverb*

A supreme love, a motive that gives a sublime rhythm to a woman's life, and exalts habit into partnership with the soul's highest needs, is not to be had where and how she wills: to know that high initiation, she must often tread where it is hard to tread, and feel the chill air, and watch through darkness.
—*George Eliot*

.

Comparing one man with another,
   You'll find this maxim true.
That the man who is good to his mother
   Will always be good to you.
—*Fred Emerson Brooks*

.

You are to me an object intensely desireable—the air I breathe in a room empty of you is unhealthy.
—*John Keats*

$\mathcal{T}$he accents of love are all that is left of
the language of paradise.
—*Edward G. Bulwer-Lytton*

•

The mind has a thousand eyes,
And the heart but one;
Yet the light of a whole life dies,
When love is done.
—*F. W. Bourdillon*

•

When you have loved as she has loved,
you grow old beautifully.
—*W. Somerset Maugham*

•

Fell in love with
A gal I thought was kind.
She made me lose ma money
An' almost lose ma mind.
—*Langston Hughes*

*T*hen while we live, in love let's so
  persevere
That when we live no more, we may
  live forever.
—*Anne Bradstreet*

.

A good marriage is that in which
each appoints the other the guardian
of his solitude.
—*Rainer Maria Rilke*

.

To love I must have something
I can put my arms around.
—*Henry Ward Beecher*

.

I love your lips when they're wet
  with wine
And red with a wicked desire.
—*Ella Wheeler Wilcox*

The couple who agrees not only to listen to each other's problems, but to make an effort to see the other side and to DO something to correct the situation is one hundred percent certain to stay out of the divorce courts.
—*Emily Post/Elizabeth L. Post*

.

If you have a friend worth loving,
Love him. Yes, and let him know
That you love him, ere life's evening
Tinge his brow with sunset glow.
—*Daniel W. Hoyt*

.

The wonderful thing about marriage is that you are the most important person in someone else's life. If you don't come home some evening, there is someone who is going to go out looking for you.
—*Dr. Joyce Brothers*

$\mathscr{T}$o love means to decide independently
to live with an equal partner, and to
subordinate oneself to the formation of a
new subject, a 'we.'
—*Fritz Kunkel*

.

The way to love anything is to realize
that it might be lost.
—*G. K. Chesterton*

.

It seemed to me pretty plain, that they
had more of love than matrimony
in them.
—*Oliver Goldsmith*

.

If love be judged by most of its visible
effects it looks more like hatred than
friendship.
—*La Rochefoucauld*

When Orpheus went down to the
      regions below,
   Which men are forbidden to see,
He tuned up his lyre, as old histories
      show,
   To set his Eurydice free.

All hell was astonished a person
      so wise
   Should rashly endanger his life,
And venture so far—but how vast
      their surprise
   When they heard that he came for
      his wife.
                    —*Thomas Lisle*

                  ·

   Was it that I went to sleep
   Thinking of him,
   That he came in my dreams?
   Had I known it a dream
   I should not have wakened.
              —*Ono Komachi*

*L*ove is the extremely difficult
realisation that something other than
oneself is real.
—*Iris Murdoch*

.

The emotion of love, in spite of the
romantics, is not self-sustaining; it
endures only when the lovers love many
things together, and not merely
each other.
—*Walter Lippmann*

.

She must know all the needs of a
    rational being,
  Be skilled to keep council, to comfort,
    to coax;
And, above all things else, be
    accomplished at seeing
  My jokes.
—*Owen Seaman*

*T*o be open to love, to trust and believe
in love, to be hopeful in love and live in
love, you need the greatest strength.
—*Leo Buscaglia*

.

In high school one learns that love
is not forever.
—*Robert Fulghum*

.

When the wind blows,
The white clouds are cleft
By the peak. Is your heart,
Like them, so cold?
—*Mibu Tadamine*

.

If two lives join, there is oft a scar,
They are one and one, with a shadowy
third;
One near one is too far.
—*Robert Browning*

*L*ove is never lost. If not reciprocated
it will flow back and soften and
purify the heart.
—*Washington Irving*

·

A man's heart is as changeable as the
skies in autumn.
A woman's heart is as changeable as the
eyes of a cat.
—*Japanese Proverbs*

·

Love is a delightful day's journey. At
the farther end kiss your companion
and say farewell.
—*Ambrose Bierce*

·

We too often love things and use people
when we should be using things and
loving people.
—*Rueul Howe*

*O*ne doesn't have to get anywhere in a marriage. It's not a public conveyance.
—*Iris Murdoch*

.

I would say that the surest measures of a man's or woman's maturity is the harmony, style, joy, dignity he creates in his marriage, and the pleasure and inspiration he provides for his spouse.
—*Benjamin Spock, M. D.*

.

Certain it is that there is no kind of affection so purely angelic as that of a father to his daughter. He beholds her both with and without regard to her sex. In love to our wives there is desire; to our sons there is ambition; but in that to our daughters there is something which there are no words to express.
—*Joseph Addison*

*S*eems lak to me de sky ain't
half so blue,
Seems lak to me dat ev'ything
wants you,
Seems lak to me I don't know
what to do,
Sence you went away.
—*James Weldon Johnson*

.

In erotic love, two people who were
separate become one. In motherly love,
two people who were one become
separate.
—*Erich Fromm*

.

I truly feel that there are as many ways
of loving as there are people in the
world and as there are days in the lives
of those people.
—*Mary Calderone*

*L*ife is short and we never have enough
time for gladdening the hearts of those
who travel the way with us. O, be
swift to love!
—*Henri F. Amiel*

.

A disappointment in love is more hard
to get over than any other; the passion
itself so softens and subdues the heart
that it disables it from struggling or
bearing up against the woes and
distresses which befall it. The mind
meets with other misfortunes in her
whole strength; she stands collected
within herself, and sustains the shock
with all the force which is natural to her;
but a heart in love has its foundation
sapped, and immediately sinks under the
weight of accidents that are disagreeable
to its favourite passion.
—*Joseph Addison*

*T*he wedding march always reminds
me of the music played when soldiers
go into battle.
—*Heinrich Heine*

.

True love is eternal, infinite, and always
like itself. It is equal and pure, without
violent demonstrations: it is seen with
white hairs and is always young
in the heart.
—*Honoré de Balzac*

.

I never could explain *why* I love
anybody, or anything.
—*Walt Whitman*

.

Loving oneself is nice but . . .
incomplete.
—*Judith Viorst*

*H*e came into my life as the warm wind
of spring had awakened flowers, as the
April showers awaken the earth. My
love for him was an unchanging love,
high and deep, free and faithful, strong
as death. Each year I learned to love
him more and more.
—*Anna Chennault*

·

Let there be spaces in your togetherness,
And let the winds of the heavens dance
between you.
—*Kahlil Gibran*

·

When I went to visit
The girl I love so much,
That winter night
The river blew so cold
That the plovers were crying.
—*Ki Tsurayuki*

*N*o cord nor cable can so forcibly draw,
or hold so fast, as love can do with a
twined thread.
—*Robert Burton*

.

'You become responsible, forever, to
what you have tamed. You are
responsible for your rose.'
—*Antoine de Saint-Exupéry*

.

Love is an expression and assertion of
self-esteem, a response to one's own
values in the person of another.
—*Ayn Rand*

.

As I listened to her voice it was as if I
were holding happiness in my hands as a
child holds up a sun-warmed apricot.
—*Llewelyn Powys*

If a man really loves a woman, of course he wouldn't marry her for the world if he were not quite sure that he was the best person she could by any possibility marry.
—*Oliver Wendell Holmes*

.

I don't know why people should feel that because they have married, they may give up all pretense of good manners and treat their partners as an 'old shoe.'
—*Emily Post/Elizabeth L. Post*

.

Far and wide, far and wide,
I can walk with you beside;

Furthermore, I tell you what,
I sit and sulk where you are not.
—*Ogden Nash*

*T*o love means to communicate to the
other that you are all for him, that you
will never fail him or let him down
when he needs you, but that you will
always be standing by with all the
necessary encouragements. It is
something one can communicate to
another only if one has it.
—*Ashley Montagu*

·

The poor cannot always reach those
whom they want to love, and they can
hardly ever escape from those whom
they no longer love.
—*E. M. Forster*

·

Love in marriage, or any close
relationship, for example, is the process
of growing hand in hand, but separately.
—*Leo Buscaglia*

*L*ove is the only satisfactory answer to
the problem of human existence.
—*Erich Fromm*

.

It is difficult to know at what moment
love begins; it is less difficult to know it
has begun. A thousand heralds proclaim
it to the listening ear, a thousand
messengers betray it to the eye. Tone,
act, attitude, and look, the signals upon
the countenance, the electric telegraph of
touch,—all these betray the yielding
citadel before the word itself is uttered,
which, like the key surrendered open
every avenue and gate of entrance, and
renders retreat impossible.
—*Henry Wadsworth Longfellow*

.

Marriage is love's demi-tasse.
—*Edgar Watson Howe*

'Yes,' I answered you last night;
'No,' this morning, sir, I say.
Colours seen by candle-light
Will not look the same by day.
—*Elizabeth Barrett Browning*

.

Love is the strange bewilderment which
overtakes one person on account of
another person.
—*James Thurber & E. B. White*

.

Jealous, *adj.* Unduly concerned about
the preservation of that which can be
lost only if not worth keeping.
—*Ambrose Bierce*

.

Hate makes us vehement partisans, but
love still more so.
—*Johann Wolfgang von Goethe*

M ore than a catbird hates a cat,
  Or a criminal hates a clue,
  Or an odalisque hates the Sultan's mates,
  That's how much I love you.
    —*Ogden Nash*

·

'A woman has got to love a bad man
once or twice in her life, to be thankful
for a good one.'
  —*Marjorie Kinnan Rawlings*

·

Sex is good, but not as good as
fresh sweet corn.
  —*Garrison Keillor*

·

I never wanted to get married. The last
thing I wanted was infinite security, and
to be the place an arrow shoots off from.
  —*Sylvia Plath*

Among those whom I like, I can find no
common denominator, but among those
whom I love, I can; all of them
make me laugh.
—W. H. Auden

.

She is so conjunctive to my life and soul
That as the star moves not but in his
sphere,
I could not but by her.
—William Shakespeare

.

In her sight there was Elysium; her smile
was heaven; her voice was enchantment;
the air of love waved round her,
breathing balm into my heart; for a little
while I had sat with the gods at their
golden tables, I had tasted of all
earth's bliss.
—William Hazlitt

After a man or woman has fallen in
love, the leaf looks better, turns of
phrase have more grace, shoulders are
more beautiful.
—*Robert Bly*

•

Absences are a good influence in love
and keep it bright and delicate.
—*Robert Louis Stevenson*

•

Give me a kiss from those sweet lips
    of thine
And make it double by enjoining mine,
Another yet, nay yet and yet another,
And let the first kiss be the second's
    brother.
Give me a thousand kisses and yet more;
And then repeat those that have gone
    before.
—*Anonymous*

What thing is love? for sure love
    is a thing.
It is a prick, it is a sting,
It is a pretty, pretty thing;
It is a fire, it is a coal,
Whose flame creeps in at every hole;
And, as my wit doth best devise,
Love's dwelling is in ladies' eyes,
From whence do glance love's piercing
    darts
That make such holes into our hearts.
       —*George Peele*

.

Never part without loving words to
think of during your absence. It may be
that you will not meet again in life.
       —*John Paul Richter*

.

Love is a great beautifier.
       —*Louisa May Alcott*

*W*hy not seize the pleasure at once? How
   often is happiness destroyed by
   preparation, foolish preparation!
               —*Jane Austen*

.

Of all the days that's in the week
   I dearly love but one day—
And that's the day that comes betwixt
   A Saturday and Monday;
For then I'm drest all in my best
   To walk abroad with Sally;
She is the darling of my heart,
   And she lives in our alley.
               —*Henry Carey*

.

I'll love you till the ocean
Is folded and hung up to dry
And the seven stars go squawking
Like geese about the sky.
               —*W. H. Auden*

$\mathcal{L}$ove is based upon a view of woman
that is impossible to any man who has
had any experience with them.
—H. L. Mencken

.

Life is a flower of which love
is the honey.
—Victor Hugo

.

To love is good; love being difficult. For
one human being to love another; that is
perhaps the most difficult of all our
tasks, the ultimate, the last test and
proof, the work for which all other
work is but preparation.
—Rainer Maria Rilke

.

Love is a hole in the heart.
—Ben Hecht

A heart as soft, a heart as kind,
  A heart as sound and free
As in the whole world thou canst find,
  That heart I'll give to thee.
      —*Robert Herrick*

·

Love is much nicer to be in than an
automobile accident, a tight girdle, a
higher tax bracket, or a holding pattern
over Philadelphia.
      —*Judith Viorst*

·

Accident counts for much in
companionship as in marriage.
      —*Henry Adams*

·

The critical period in matrimony is
breakfast-time.
      —*A. P. Herbert*

*S*oon—in a few months, perhaps, my angel will sleep in my arms, will awaken in my arms, will live there. All your thoughts at all moments, all your looks will be for me; all my thoughts, all my moments, all my looks, will be for you!
—*Victor Hugo*

.

Friendship is a disinterested commerce between equals; love, an abject intercourse between tyrants and slaves.
—*Oliver Goldsmith*

.

Miss Manners has always subscribed to the romantic notion that love is erratic and inexplicable, and that the most sensible matching of requirements is no more likely to produce it than differences are to discourage it.
—*Judith Martin (Miss Manners)*

*T*he best part about married life is the
fights. The rest is merely so-so.
—*Thornton Wilder*

•

The very fact that we make such a to-do
over golden weddings indicates our
amazement at human endurance. The
celebration is more in the nature of a
reward for stamina.
—*Ilka Chase*

•

Whilst Adam slept, Eve from his
side arose:
Strange his first sleep should be his
last repose.
—*Anonymous*

•

Love rules his kingdom without a sword.
—*English Proverb*

$\mathcal{I}$t is easy to reconcile when there is love.
　　　—*Welsh Proverb*

．

And what is bettre than wisedoom?
　　Womman.
And what is bettre than a good
　　womman?
Nothyng.
　　　　—*Geoffrey Chaucer*

．

I am a lover and have not found my
　　thing to love.
　　　—*Sherwood Anderson*

．

All that a man has to say or do that can
possibly concern mankind, is in some
shape or other to tell the story of his
love—to sing and, if he is fortunate and
keeps alive, he will be forever in love.
　　　—*Henry David Thoreau*

I hated that woman because she did not make you happy, but I would have hated her a hundred times more if you had been happy with her. I thought she had robbed me of what should be mine only, what is my right, because I love you more than anyone and value you above everything in the world.
—*Nadejda Philaretovna von Meck*

.

Love! thou hast every bliss in store;
'Tis friendship, and 'tis something more;
Each other every wish they give:
Not to know love is not to live.
—*John Gay*

.

Hatred paralyzes life; love releases it.
Hatred confuses life; love harmonizes it.
Hatred darkens life; love illumines it.
—*Martin Luther King, Jr.*

*L*ove is not in our choice, but
in our fate.
—*John Dryden*

.

Love lives in cottages as well as
in courts.
—*English Proverb*

.

Fair is the white star of twilight,
And the sky clearer
At the day's end;
But she is fairer, and she is dearer
She, my heart's friend!

Fair is the white star of twilight,
And the moon roving
To the sky's end;
But she is fairer, better worth loving,
She, my heart's friend.
—*Shoshone Song (Mary Austin, tr.)*

*W*e love a girl for very different things than understanding. We love her for her beauty, her youth, her mirth, her confidingness, her character, with its faults, caprices, and God knows what other inexpressible charms; but we do not love her understanding. Her mind we esteem if it is brilliant, and it may greatly elevate her in our opinion; nay, more, it may enchain us when we already love. But her understanding is not that which awakens and inflames our passions.
—*Johann Wolfgang von Goethe*

.

'Summer is coming, summer is coming,
   I know it, I know it, I know it.
Light again, leaf again, life again, love
   again,'
Yes, my wild little Poet.
      —*Alfred, Lord Tennyson*

*L*ove me, lady, dearly,
 If you'll be so good;
Though I don't see clearly
 On what ground you should.
  —*C. S. Calverley*

.

No man is in love when he marries. He
 may have loved before; I have even
heard he has sometimes loved after: but
at the time never. There is something in
 the formalities of the matrimonial
 preparations that drive away all
  the little cupidons.
   —*Fanny Burney*

.

My form, my friends observe with pain,
 Is growing daily thinner.
Love only occupies the brain
 That once could think of dinner.
  —*P. G. Wodehouse*

Should poets bicycle-pump the human
    heart
Or squash it flat?
Man's love is of man's life a thing apart;
Girls aren't like that.
        —*Kingsley Amis*

·

Bride, n. A woman with a fine prospect
    of happiness behind her.
        —*Ambrose Bierce*

·

Good communication is as stimulating as
    black coffee, and just as hard
        to sleep after.
        —*Anne Morrow Lindbergh*

·

A honeymoon is a good deal like a man
laying off to take an expensive vacation,
    and coming back to a different job.
        —*Edgar Watson Howe*

When I was planting young apple trees and pear trees, I cut the name of my dearest on the bark. Since, there has been no end or peace to my passion: as the tree grows, my love glows; the heart gives body to the letters.
—*Florus*

.

Will you give me yourself? will you come travel with me?
Shall we stick by each other as long as we live?
—*Walt Whitman*

.

A man reserves his greatest and deepest love not for the woman in whose company he finds himself electrified and enkindled but for that one in whose company he may feel tenderly drowsy.
—*George Jean Nathan*

*Y*oung love is a flame; very pretty, often very hot and fierce, but still only light and flickering. The love of the older and disciplined heart is as coals, deep-burning, unquenchable.
—*Henry Ward Beecher*

.

Some men, some men
Cannot pass a
Crap game.
(He said he'd come at moonrise, and
    here's another day!)
    —*Dorothy Parker*

.

I don't care
   if you desert me.
Many pretty boys are in the town.
Soon I shall take another one.
That is not hard for me!
    —*Chinook Song*

*L*ove is just a system for getting someone to call you darling after sex.
—*Julian Barnes*

·

The greatest comfort, when one is rejected, is to believe that the other person is making a mistake, which will be bitterly regretted sooner or later.
—*Judith Martin (Miss Manners)*

·

Literature is mostly about having sex and not much about having children. Life is the other way round.
—*David Lodge*

·

'Do you think it is ever possible to be successful in love, if one doesn't make an effort to help things along?'
—*Marguerite Duras*

I want (who does not want?) a wife
   Affectionate and fair,
To solace all the woes of life
   And all its days to share;
Of temper sweet, of yielding will,
   Of firm yet placid mind,
With all my faults to love me still,
   With sentiments refined.
      —*John Quincy Adams*

.

Love is the 'crazy glue' that holds a
couple together and strengthens the
   relationship year after year.
      —*Dr. Joyce Brothers*

.

I once was a maid, tho' I cannot
   tell when,
And still my delight is in proper
   young men.
      —*Robert Burns*

*B*ehind every man who achieves
    success
Stand a mother, a wife and the IRS.
        —Ethel Jacobson

·

If young women do not wish to appear
coquettish, if elderly men do not wish to
be ridiculous, they should never refer to
love as something with which they could
be personally concerned.
        —La Rochefoucauld

·

Love has ceased to be the rather fearful,
mysterious thing it was, and become a
perfectly normal, almost commonplace,
activity—an activity, for many young
people especially in America, of the same
nature as dancing or tennis, a sport, a
recreation, a pastime.
        —Aldous Huxley

*L*ove is merely madness; and I tell you
deserves as well a dark house and a
whip, as madmen do; and the reason
why they are not so punished and cured,
is that the lunacy is so ordinary, that the
whippers are in love too.
—*William Shakespeare*

·

Difficult or easy, pleasant or bitter, you
are the same you: I cannot live with
you—or without you.
—*Martial*

·

She is not fair to outward view
As many maidens be;
Her loveliness I never knew
Until she smiled on me.
Oh! then I saw her eye was bright,
A well of love, a spring of light.
—*Hartley Coleridge*

$\mathscr{A}$ll other things, to their destruction
     draw,
Only our love hath no decay;
This no tomorrow hath, nor yesterday,
Running it never runs from us away,
But truly keeps his first, last, everlasting
     day.
                    —*John Donne*

.

Don't wish me happiness—I don't
expect to be happy, but it's gotten
beyond that, somehow. Wish me
courage and strength and a sense of
humor—I will need them all.
          —*Anne Morrow Lindbergh*

.

A man always remembers his first love
with special tenderness. But after that he
begins to bunch them.
          —*H. L. Mencken*

*E*ver has it been that love knows not its own depth until the hour of separation.
—*Kahlil Gibran*

.

When you fish for love, bait with your heart, not your brain.
—*Mark Twain*

.

There is a comfort in the strength
  of love;
'Twill make a thing endurable,
  which else
Would overset the brain, or break
  the heart.
—*William Wordsworth*

.

The entire sum of existence is the magic of being needed by just one person.
—*Vi Putnam*

*W*e complete ourselves. If we haven't
the power to complete ourselves, the
search for love becomes a search for
self-annihilation; and then we try
to convince ourselves that
self-annihilation is love.
—*Erica Jong*

.

In friendship, as in love, we are often
happier because of the things we do not
know than because of those we know.
—*La Rochefoucauld*

.

It's clear what Bob and I both need:
a *wife!*
—*Jane Wagner*

.

Sex alleviates tension. Love causes it.
—*Woody Allen*

I should like to know what is the proper function of women, if it is not to make reasons for husbands to stay at home, and still stronger reasons for bachelors to go out.
—*George Eliot*

.

For talk six times with the same single lady,
And you may get the wedding dresses ready.
—*Lord Byron*

.

The accepted and betrothed lover has lost the wildest charm of his maiden in her acceptance of him. She was heaven while he pursued her as a star, she cannot be heaven if she stoops to such a one as he.
—*Ralph Waldo Emerson*

*L*ove is like the measles; we all
have to go through it.
—*Jerome K. Jerome*

.

She must see if she really *wants* you,
wants to keep you and to have no other
man all her life. It means forfeiting
something. But the only principle I can
see in this life, is that one *must* forfeit
the less for the greater. Only one must
be thoroughly honest about it.
—*D. H. Lawrence*

.

Julia, I bring
To thee this ring,
    Made for thy finger fit;
To show by this
That our love is
    Or should be, like to it.
—*Robert Herrick*

*I*n all thy humours, whether
    grave or mellow,
Thou'rt such a touchy, testy,
    pleasant fellow;
Hast so much wit, and mirth, and
    spleen about thee,
There is no living with thee, nor
    without thee.
    —*Joseph Addison*

.

Man and woman are two locked
caskets, of which each contains the
    key to the other.
    —*Isak Dinesen*

.

For lover's eyes more sharp-sighted be
Than other men's, and in dear love's
    sight
See more than any other eyes can see.
    —*Edmund Spenser*

*I*t should be of the pleasure of a poem itself to tell how it can. The figure a poem makes. It begins in delight and ends in wisdom. The figure is the same as for love.
—*Robert Frost*

·

It is possible that a man can be so changed by love that one could not recognize him as the same person.
—*Terence*

·

True Love is but a humble, low-born thing,
And hath its food served up in earthen ware;
It is a thing to walk with, hand in hand,
Through the everydayness of this workaday world.
—*James Russell Lowell*

$\mathcal{T}$he science of love is the philosophy
of the heart.
—*Cicero*

.

Here I sit on this point, whence I can
see the man that I love.
Our people think that they can sever us;
but I shall see him while the world
lasts.
Here shall I remain, in sight of the
one I love.
—*Abanaki Song*

.

All love at first, like generous wine,
Ferments and frets, until 'tis fine;
But when 'tis settled on the lee,
And from th' impurer matter free,
Becomes the richer still, the older,
And proves the pleasanter, the colder.
—*Samuel Butler*

*Y*esterday I loved, today I suffer,
tomorrow I die: but I still think fondly,
today and tomorrow, of yesterday.
—*G. E. Lessing*

.

Love makes time pass away, and time
makes love pass away.
—*French Proverb*

.

Love keeps the cold out better than a
cloak. It serves for food and raiment.
—*Henry Wadsworth Longfellow*

.

Is it so small a thing
To have enjoyed the sun,
To have lived light in the spring,
To have loved, to have thought,
to have done.
—*Matthew Arnold*

*I*t would be a fine thing, just the same, in which I hardly dare believe, to pass our lives near each other, hypnotized by our dreams: *your* patriotic dream, *our* humanitarian dream and *our* scientific dream.
—*Pierre Curie*

.

How do I love thee? Let me count the ways.
—*Elizabeth Barrett Browning*

.

Happiness makes up in height for what it lacks in length.
—*Robert Frost*

.

He who says o'er much 'I love not' is in love.
—*Ovid*

*S*o you, that are the sovereign of my
  heart,
Have all my joys attending on your will:
My joys low ebbing when you do
  depart,
When you return, their tide my heart
  doth fill.
　　　　　—*Charles Best*

·

Dear Marilyn:
Why are some men so smart, neat,
caring, and helpful—until they become
husbands?
　　　　　—*Anonymous*
　　　　　Richmond, Virginia

Dear Reader:
Probably for the same reason that some
women are so smart, neat, caring, and
helpful until they become wives.
　　　　　—*Marilyn vos Savant*

*S*ing, for faith and hope are high—
More so true as you and I—
Sing the Lovers' Litany;
'Love like ours can never die!'
—*Rudyard Kipling*

·

The love of a mother is never exhausted,
it never changes, it never tires. A father
may turn his back on his child, brothers
and sisters may become inveterate
enemies, husbands may desert their
wives, wives their husbands. But a
mother's love endures through all.
—*Washington Irving*

·

I who employ a poet's tongue,
Would tell you how
You are a golden damson hung
Upon a silver bough.
—*Countee Cullen*

From quiet homes and first beginning,
Out to the undiscovered ends,
There's nothing worth the wear of
    winning,
But laughter and the love of friends.
    —*Hilaire Belloc*

.

Grown children come home when they
are out of work, out of sorts, out of
money, or out of love.
    —*Erma Bombeck*

.

Absence lessens moderate passions and
intensifies great ones, as the wind blows
out a candle but fans up a fire.
    —*La Rochefoucauld*

.

Love is a ring, and a ring has no end.
    —*Russian Proverb*

*S*hall I tell you what makes love so dangerous? 'Tis the too high idea we are apt to form of it. But to speak the truth, love, considered as a passion, is merely a blind instinct, that we should rate accordingly. It is an appetite, which inclines us to one object, rather than another, without our being able to account for our taste.
—*Ninon de l'Enclos*

.

The glory of the day was in her face,
The beauty of the night was in her eyes.
And over all her loveliness, the grace
Of Morning blushing in the early skies.
—*James Weldon Johnson*

.

If you marry, you will regret it. If you do not marry, you will also regret it.
—*Søren Kierkegaard*

*I*t isn't possible to love and to part.
You will wish that it was. You can
transmute love, ignore it, muddle it, but
you can never pull it out of you.
—*E. M. Forster*

.

Truth, that's brighter than gem,
Trust, that's purer than pearl—
Brightest truth, purest trust in the
universe—
All were for me in the kiss of
one girl.
—*Robert Browning*

.

Brigham Young has two hundred
wives. . . . He loves not wisely but two
hundred well. He is dreadfully married.
He's the most married man I ever
saw in my life.
—*Artemus Ward*

*S*ome luck lies in not getting what you thought you wanted but getting what you have, which once you have it you may be smart enough to see is what you would have wanted had you known.
—*Garrison Keillor*

·

Why is it no one ever sent me yet
    One perfect limousine, do you
        suppose?
Ah no, it's always just my luck to get
    One perfect rose.
            —*Dorothy Parker*

·

I love you, and you love me,—at least, you *say so*, and *act* as if you *did* so, which last is a great consolation in all events. But *I* more than love you, and cannot cease to love you.
            —*Lord Byron*

*M*oney, it turned out, was exactly like sex, you thought of nothing else if you didn't have it and thought of other things if you did.
—*James Baldwin*

·

When once a woman has given you her heart, you can never get rid of the rest of her body.
—*John Vanbrugh*

·

Women are really much nicer than men: No wonder we like them.
—*Kingsley Amis*

·

The heart *prefers* to move against the grain of circumstance; perversity is the soul's very life.
—*John Updike*

*K*now when *not* to compete. You could have any one of a number of fascinating men, but you've decided you want Robert Redford. This isn't a realistic goal for several reasons: 1) He's taken. 2) The chances of your meeting him are not very good. 3) Are you sure you could really *stand* being married to a movie star?
—*Nancy Winters*

.

With children no longer the universally accepted reason for marriage, marriages are going to have to exist on their own merits.
—*Eleanor Holmes Norton*

.

We love the things we love in spite of what they are.
—*Louis Untermeyer*

*W*e cannot permit love to run riot;
we must build fences around it, as
we do around pigs.
—*Edgar Watson Howe*

.

There are no words so fine, no flattery
so soft, that there is not a sentiment
beyond them, that it is impossible to
express, at the bottom of the heart
where true love is.
—*William Hazlitt*

.

Do not marry your lover, and never take
back the man you have divorced.
—*Lebanese Proverb*

.

Love and scandal are the best
sweeteners of tea.
—*Henry Fielding*

A mother's love!
  If there be one thing pure,
  Where all beside is sullied,
  That can endure,
  When all else passes away;
  If there be aught
Surpassing human deed or word, or
      thought,
    It is a mother's love.
      —*Marchioness de Spadara*

·

To love is to place our happiness in the
      happiness of another.
      —*G. W. Leibnitz*

·

But love me for love's sake, that
      evermore
  Thou mayest love on, through love's
  eternity.
      —*Elizabeth Barrett Browning*

*M*y chief occupation, despite
appearances, has always been love. I
have a romantic soul, and have always
had considerable trouble interesting
it in something else.
—*Albert Camus*

.

Romance cannot be put into quantity
production—the moment love becomes
casual, it becomes commonplace.
—*Frederick Lewis Allen*

.

Love is a mutual self-giving which
ends in self-recovery.
—*Bishop Fulton J. Sheen*

.

Happiness is having a large, loving,
caring, close-knit family in another city.
—*George Burns*

*Y*ou mustn't force sex to do the work of love or love to do the work of sex.
—*Mary McCarthy*

.

Love is the strongest force the world possesses, and yet it is the humblest imaginable.
—*Mahatma Gandhi*

.

There is no surprise more magical than the surprise of being loved. It is the finger of God on a man's shoulder.
—*Charles Morgan*

.

What men call gallantry, and gods adultery,
Is much more common where the climate's sultry.
—*Lord Byron*

When he shall die,
Take him and cut him out in little stars,
And he will make the face of heaven
     so fine
That all the world will be in love
     with night.
                    —*William Shakespeare*

.

That which is loved is always beautiful.
                    —*Norwegian Proverb*

.

All, everything that I understand, I
     understand only because I love.
                    —*Leo Tolstoy*

.

Love's of a strangely open simple kind,
And thinks none see it 'cause itself is
     blind.
                    —*Abraham Cowley*

*M*arriage involves big compromises
all the time. International-level
compromises. You're the U.S.A., he's
the USSR, and you're talking
nuclear warheads.
—*Bette Midler*

.

Daphne knows, with equal ease,
How to vex and how to please,
But the folly of her sex
Makes her sole delight to vex.
—*Jonathan Swift*

.

There is a big deposit of sympathy in the
bank of love, but don't draw out little
sums every hour or two—so that by and
by, when perhaps you need it badly, it is
all drawn out and you yourself don't
know how or on what it was spent.
—*Emily Post/Elizabeth L. Post*

*M*arriage is a wonderful invention; but,
then again, so is a bicycle repair kit.
—*Billy Connolly*

·

Old bachelors and old maids are either
too good or too bad.
—*Basque Proverb*

·

In recent years it has become common
to hear people all over the country speak
of long-term marriage in a tone of voice
that assumes it to be inextricably
intertwined with the music of
Lawrence Welk.
—*Calvin Trillin*

·

It would have been a wonderful
wedding—had it not been mine.
—*Erma Bombeck*

A mighty pain to love it is
And 'tis a pain that pain to miss
But of all pains the greatest pain
It is to love and love in vain.
—*Abraham Cowley*

.

If only one could tell true love from
false love as one can tell mushrooms
from toadstools.
—*Katherine Mansfield*

.

'Do you want me to tell you something
really subversive? Love *is* everything it's
cracked up to be. That's why people are
so cynical about it.'
—*Erica Jong*

.

There's a book in every marriage.
—*Erma Bombeck*

I feel that all disease is ultimately related to a lack of love, or to love that is only conditional, for the exhaustion and depression of the immune system thus created leads to physical vulnerability. I also feel that all healing is related to the ability to give and accept unconditional love.
—*Bernie S. Siegel, M. D.*

.

It warms me, it charms me,
  To mention but her name;
It heats me, it beats me,
  And set me a' on flame.
—*Robert Burns*

.

To find yourself jilted is a blow to your pride. Do your best to forget it and if you don't succeed, at least pretend to.
—*Molière*

*M*arriage is not just spiritual communion and passionate embraces; marriage is also three-meals-a-day and remembering to carry out the trash.
—*Dr. Joyce Brothers*

.

My husband wanted to live in sin, even *after* we were married.
—*James Thurber*

.

Love's supreme miracle is to cure coquetry.
—*La Rochefoucauld*

.

Woman, though so kind she seems, will take your heart and tantalize it,
Were it made of Portland stone, she'd manage to McAdamize it.
—*James Planché*

*H*ear the mellow wedding bells,—
    Golden bells!
What a world of happiness their
    harmony foretells!
      —*Edgar Allan Poe*

.

A man should be taller, older, heavier,
uglier, and hoarser than his wife.
      —*Edgar Watson Howe*

.

Quoth he, to bid me not to love,
Is to forbid my pulse to move,
My beard to grow, my ears to prick up,
Or (when I'm in a fit) to hiccup.
      —*Samuel Butler*

.

Love and hunger are the foundation
    stones of all things.
      —*Russian Proverb*

*T*here is not one in a hundred of
either sex who is not taken in when
they marry.
—*Jane Austen*

.

He must walk—like a god of old story
  Come down from the home of his
    rest;
He must smile—like the sun in his glory
  On the buds he loves ever the best;
And oh! from its ivory portal
  Like music his soft speech must
    flow!—
If he speak, smile, or walk like a mortal,
  My own Araminta, say 'No!'
—*W. M. Praed*

.

In married life, three is company
and two is none.
—*Oscar Wilde*

*B*y god, D. H. Lawrence was right when he had said there must be a dumb, dark, dull, bitter belly-tension between a man and a woman, and how else could this be achieved save in the long monotony of marriage?
—*Stella Gibbons*

·

One good Husband is worth two good Wives; for the scarcer things are, the more they're valued.
—*Benjamin Franklin*

·

Among all the many kinds of first love, that which begins in childish companionship is the strongest and most enduring; when passion comes to unite its force to long affection, love is at its spring-tide.
—*George Eliot*

*J*oy is a net of love by which
you can catch souls.
—*Mother Teresa*

.

It is only with the heart that one
can see rightly; what is essential is
invisible to the eye.
—*Antoine de Saint-Exupéry*

.

Love is not to be reason'd down or lost
In high ambition, or a thirst of greatness;
'Tis second life; it grows into the soul
Warms ev'ry vein, and beats in ev'ry
pulse.
—*Joseph Addison*

.

Love, cough, and a smoke, can't
well be hid.
—*Benjamin Franklin*

A crowd is not company, and faces are but a gallery of pictures, and talk but a tinkling cymbal, where there is no love.
—*Francis Bacon*

.

If a family has an old person in it, it possesses a jewel.
—*Chinese Proverb*

.

But Love, at least, is not a state
Either *en vogue* or out-of-date.
—*W. H. Auden*

.

That is the true season of love, when we believe that we alone can love, that no one could ever have loved so before us, and that no one will love in the same way after us.
—*Johann Wolfgang von Goethe*

What the world needs is not romantic lovers who are sufficient unto themselves, but husbands and wives who live in communities, relate to other people, carry on useful work and willingly give time and attention to their children.
—*Margaret Mead*

.

The car, the furniture, the wife, the children—everything has to be disposable. Because you see the main thing today is—shopping.
—*Arthur Miller*

.

Children of the future Age
Reading this indignant page,
Know that in a former time
Love! sweet Love! was thought a crime.
—*William Blake*

*I*n love there are two things:
    bodies and words.
        —*Joyce Carol Oates*

.

Now that I have your heart by heart,
    I see.
        —*Louise Bogan*

.

Love is woman's moon and sun;
Man has other forms of fun.
        —*Dorothy Parker*

.

The master, the swabber, the boatswain
    and I,
    The gunner and his mate,
Loved Mall, Meg, and Marian and
    Margery.
But none of us cared for Kate.
        —*William Shakespeare*

*I*t took me longer to win Camille's parents than it had taken me to win her; but finally I broke them down and made them realize that Camille could be happy marrying beneath her.
—*Bill Cosby*

.

Bigamy is having one husband too many. Monogamy is the same.
—*Erica Jong*

.

Love has the quality of informing almost everything—even one's work.
—*Sylvia Ashton-Warner*

.

Those who have known great passions remain all through their lives both glad and sorry they have recovered.
—*La Rochefoucauld*

The allurement that women hold out to men is precisely the allurement that Cape Hatteras holds out to sailors: they are enormously dangerous and hence enormously fascinating.
—*H. L. Mencken*

.

Love is the perpetual source of fears and anxieties.
—*Ovid*

.

Brute, *n.* SEE HUSBAND.
Husband, *n.* One who, having dined, is charged with the care of the plate.
—*Ambrose Bierce*

.

Good marriages do exist, but not delectable ones.
—*La Rochefoucauld*

*W*e owe to the Middle Ages the two worst inventions of humanity—romantic love and gunpowder.
—*André Maurois*

.

Beauty, *n*. The power by which a woman charms a lover and terrifies a husband.
—*Ambrose Bierce*

.

You know what charm is: a way of getting the answer yes without having asked any clear question.
—*Albert Camus*

.

You, that are going to be married, think things can never be done too fast; but we, that are old, and know what we are about, must elope methodically, madam.
—*Oliver Goldsmith*

The essence of a good marriage is respect for each other's personality combined with that deep intimacy, physical, mental, and spiritual, which makes a serious love between man and woman the most fructifying of all human experiences.
—*Bertrand Russell*

.

You, because you love me, hold
Fast to me, caress me, be
Quiet and kind, comfort me
With stillness, say nothing at all.
—*Kenneth Rexroth*

.

When a person is in love, he seems to himself wholly changed from what he was before; and he fancies that everybody sees him in the same light.
—*Blaise Pascal*

*I*f the heart of a man is depress'd
    with cares,
The mist is dispell'd when a woman
    appears;
Like the notes of a fiddle, she sweetly,
    sweetly
Raises the spirits, and charms our ears,
Roses and lilies her cheeks disclose,
But her ripe lips are more sweet
    than those.
Press her,
Caress her,
With blisses,
Her kisses
Dissolve us in pleasure and soft repose.
    —*John Gay*

.

I am Tarzan of the Apes. I want you. I
am yours. You are mine. We will live
here together always in my house.
    —*Edgar Rice Burroughs*

*T*he man who thinks he loves a woman
for her own sake is very much mistaken.
—*La Rochefoucauld*

·

Marriage and cooking call for
forethought.
—*Greek Proverb*

·

To love you have to learn to understand
the other, more than she understands
herself, and to submit to her
understanding of you. It is damnably
difficult and painful, but it is the only
thing which endures.
—*D. H. Lawrence*

·

Men and women, women and men.
It will never work.
—*Erica Jong*

How do you know love is gone? If you said that you would be there at seven and you get there by nine, and he or she has not called the police yet—it's gone.
—*Marlene Dietrich*

.

Never marry but for love; but see that thou lovest what is lovely.
—*William Penn*

.

Love doesn't just sit there, like a stone, it has to be made, like bread; re-made all the time, made new.
—*Ursula Le Guin*

.

The most powerful symptom of love is a tenderness which becomes at times almost insupportable.
—*Victor Hugo*

*F*ound while spring-cleaning
　But too precious to throw out,
　The first love's letters.
　　　　—Anonymous

·

A woman is more considerate in affairs
of love than a man; because love is more
　the study and business of her life.
　　　　—Washington Irving

·

Is this a kind of loving too,
a chocolate bar that tastes good at
　　the time
but kills the dinner later on?
　　　　—Rod McKuen

·

Love and eggs should be fresh
　　to be enjoyed.
　　　　—Russian Proverb

*D*on't you think I was made for you? I feel like you had me ordered—and I was delivered to you—to be worn—I want you to wear me, like a watch-charm or a button hole boquet [*sic*]—to the world.
—*Zelda Fitzgerald*

.

Come, let's be a comfortable couple and take care of each other! How glad we shall be, that we have somebody we are fond of always, to talk to and sit with.
—*Charles Dickens*

.

God be thanked, the meanest of
   his creatures
Boasts two soul-sides, one to face
   the world with,
One to show a woman when he
   loves her!
—*Robert Browning*

If I had had a pistol I would have shot
  him—either that or fallen at his feet.
There is no middle way when one loves.
        —*Lady Troubridge*

.

All men to some one quality incline:
Only to love is naturally mine.
        —*Michael Drayton*

.

Life without love's a load, and
    time stands still;
What we refuse to him, to death
    we give:
And then then only when we love
    we live.
        —*William Congreve*

.

Love comforteth like sunshine after rain.
        —*William Shakespeare*

True love can no more be diminished by showers of evil-hap, than flowers are marred by timely rains.
—*Sir Philip Sidney*

.

Noble birth will be of no avail to you in love: Cupid is not impressed by family portraits.
—*Propertius*

.

Love is a canvas furnished by Nature and embroidered by imagination.
—*Voltaire*

.

Full as an egg was I with glee,
    And happy as a king.
Good Lord! how all men envied me!
    She loved like anything.
—*John Gay*

*W*omen speak because they wish to speak, whereas a man speaks only when driven to speech by something outside himself—like, for instance, he can't find any clean socks.
—*Jean Kerr*

.

But a smooth and steadfast mind,
    Gentle thoughts, and calm desires,
Hearts with equal love combined,
    Kindle never-dying fires:—
Where these are not, I despise
Lovely cheeks or lips or eyes.
—*Thomas Carew*

.

No stranger can get a great many notes of torture out of a human soul; it takes one that knows it well—parent, child, brother, sister, intimate.
—*Oliver Wendell Holmes*

$\mathscr{L}$ove is not altogether a delirium, yet it has many points in common therewith. I call it rather a discerning of the infinite in the finite—of the ideal made real.
—*Thomas Carlyle*

.

There are two sound reasons for making up at bedtime: it feels like the right moment for reconciliation and a fight is harder to sustain when one of the fighters falls asleep.
—*Bill Cosby*

.

My love for Linton is like the foliage in the woods; time will change it, I'm well aware, as winter changes the trees—My love for Heathcliff resembles the eternal rocks beneath:—a source of little visible delight, but necessary.
—*Emily Brontë*

*I*n the presence of someone who has been married a long time to the same person, a lot of people seem to feel the way they might feel in the presence of a Methodist clergyman or an IRS examiner.
—*Calvin Trillin*

·

Every human being, my dear, must be viewed according to what it is good for, for none of us, no, not one, is perfect; and were we to love none who had imperfections, this would be a desert for our love.
—*Thomas Jefferson*

·

Rub your eyes and purify your heart and prize above all else in the world those who love you and who wish you well.
—*Aleksandr Solzhenitsyn*

*W*ild Nights—Wild Nights!
   Were I with thee
   Wild Nights should be
   Our luxury!
       —*Emily Dickinson*

.

Love is a pearl of purest hue,
   But stormy waves are round it;
And dearly may a woman rue,
   The house that first she found it.
       —*L. E. Landon*

.

No matter how old our daughters are,
we still ache and dream for them.
       —*Lois Wyse*

.

There is a time for work. And a time for
love. That leaves no other time.
       —*Coco Chanel*

*N*othing in the world is single;
All things by a law divine
In one another's being mingle;
Why not I with thine?
—*Percy Bysshe Shelley*

.

God has a peculiar right over the hearts
of great men He has created. When He
pleases to touch them He ravishes them,
and lets them not speak nor breathe but
for His glory. Till that moment of grace
arrives, O think of me—do not forget
me—remember my love and fidelity and
constancy: love me as your mistress,
cherish me as your child, your sister,
your wife!
—*Heloise*

.

Never go to bed mad. Stay up and fight.
—*Phyllis Diller*

A successful marriage requires falling
in love many times, always with the
same person.
—*Mignon McLaughlin*

.

You ask me, sweetheart, to avow
   What charm in you I most adore,
But how can I discriminate
   From your innumerable store.
—*George Roberts*

.

There is no more lovely, friendly, and
charming relationship, communion, or
company than a good marriage.
—*Martin Luther*

.

Your words are my food, your breath
my wine. You are everything to me.
—*Sarah Bernhardt*

To the partial eyes of a lover, pockmarks
seem like dimples.
—*Japanese Proverb*

.

If to her share some female errors fall,
Look on her face, and you'll forget
'em all.
—*Alexander Pope*

.

'I hope I'm doing the right thing' he
thought looking in the mirror, 'Am I
good enough for her?' Roger need not
have worried because he was
—*John Lennon*

.

The good or ill hap of a good or ill life,
is the good or ill choice of a good
or ill wife.
—*Benjamin Franklin*

*P*ains of love be sweeter far
Than all other pleasures are.
—*John Dryden*

.

Although we women are always assumed
to be the romantics of the world, it is
oftentimes men who are romantic and
women who are pragmatic.
—*Lois Wyse*

.

The love we give away is the only
love we keep.
—*Elbert Hubbard*

.

When a woman gets married, it's like
jumping into a hole in the ice in the
middle of winter: you do it once and
you remember it the rest of your days.
—*Maxim Gorky*

I want to die while you love me,
While yet you hold me fair,
While laughter lies upon my lips
And lights are in my hair.
—*Georgia Douglas Johnson*

.

I looked only for goodness of heart, an
ingenuous and affectionate disposition,
a good understanding, etc., and the
character of my wife is too frank and
single-hearted to suffer me to fear that I
may be disappointed. I do myself wrong;
I did not look for these nor any other
qualities, but they trapped me before I
was aware, and now I am married in
spite of myself.
—*William Cullen Bryant*

.

Speak low if you speak love.
—*William Shakespeare*

*B*e to her virtues very kind.
Be to her faults a little blind.
—*Matthew Prior*

.

The world well tried—the sweetest thing
in life
Is the unclouded welcome of a wife.
—*Nathaniel Parker Willis*

.

This to the Crown, and blessing of
my life,
The much lov'd husband, of a happy
wife.
—*Anne Finch*

.

I hope before long to crush you in my
arms and cover you with a million kisses
burning as though beneath the equator.
—*Napoleon Bonaparte*